HOW TO
TOLERATE
LACTOSE
INTOLERANCE

HOW TO TOLERATE LACTOSE INTOLERANCE

Recipes & A Guide for Eating Well Without Dairy Products

by

Phyllis Z. Goldberg, R.D.H., B.A.

West Hartford, Connecticut

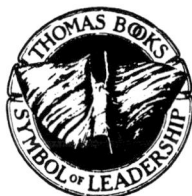

CHARLES C THOMAS • PUBLISHER, LTD.
Springfield • Illinois • U.S.A.

Published and Distributed Throughout the World by

CHARLES C THOMAS • PUBLISHER, LTD.
2600 South First Street
Springfield, Illinois 62794-9265

© *1998 by* CHARLES C THOMAS • PUBLISHER, LTD.
ISBN 0-398-06869-0

Library of Congress Catalog Card Number: 98-3438

With THOMAS BOOKS *careful attention is given to all details of manufacturing
and design. It is the Publisher's desire to present books that are satisfactory as to their
physical qualities and artistic possibilities and appropriate for their particular use.*
THOMAS BOOKS *will be true to those laws of quality that assure a good name
and good will.*

Printed in the United States of America
CR-R-3

Library of Congress Cataloging in Publication Data

Goldberg, Phyllis Z.
    How to tolerate lactose intolerance : recipes and a guide for
eating well without dairy products / by Phyllis Z. Goldberg.
        p.   cm.
    Includes bibliographical references and index.
    ISBN 0-398-06869-0 (paper)
    1. Lactose intolerance--Diet therapy--Recipes. 2. Milk-free diet-
-Recipes. I. Title.
RC632.L33G65   1998
616.3'998--dc21   98-3438
                                                                        CIP

To my family and to my husband Mort, my hero,
for his encouragement and support, but most especially for his love,
lo these many years.

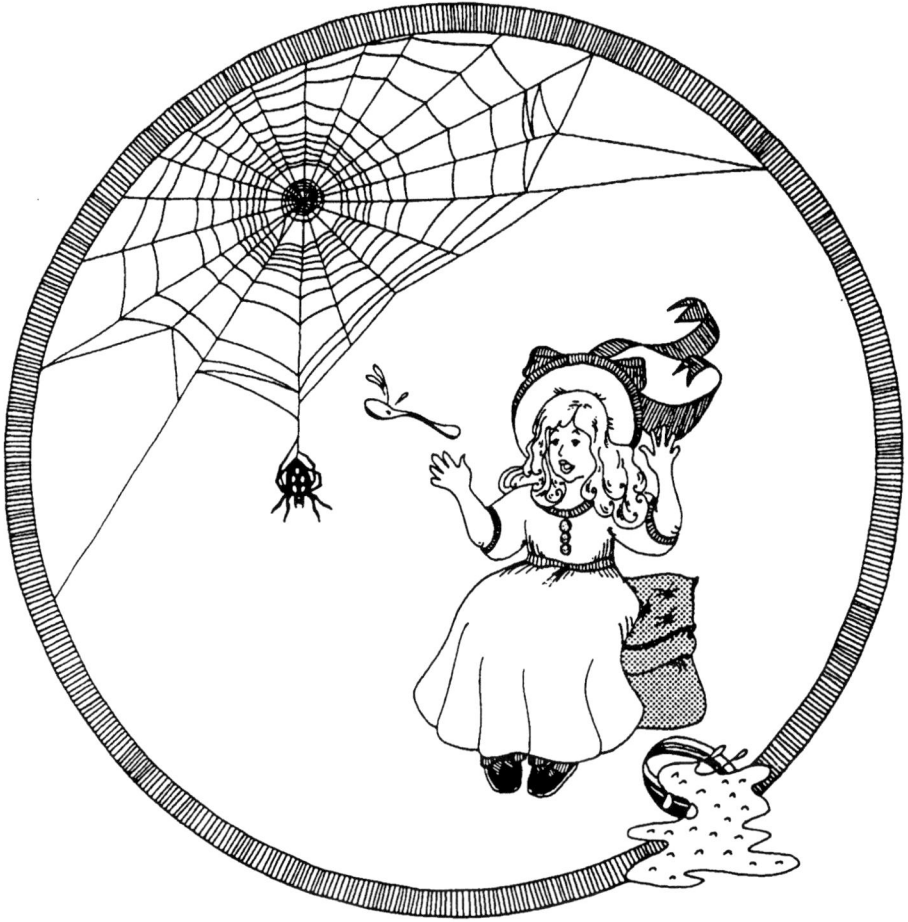

Little Miss Muffet sat on a tuffet
Eating her curds and whey;
There came a great spider
Who sat down beside her
And frightened Miss Muffet away.

FOREWORD

Lactose intolerance is extremely common. Nearly 50 million Americans have lactose intolerance. Lactase, the enzyme that digests lactose (the sugar in milk), diminishes in activity as one ages. Symptoms of lactose intolerance such as gas, bloating, abdominal pain, and diarrhea usually occur within two hours of the ingestion of milk. These symptoms begin to develop in the teenage and young adult population. If one becomes lactose intolerant, the symptoms may increase with age.

The enzyme lactase is produced in the small intestine. It breaks down milk sugar so that it can be absorbed from the small intestine into blood vessels. Lactose cannot be absorbed without lactase. For reasons that are not yet clearly understood, less lactase is produced with aging. When the amount of lactase decreases to a certain critical level, the symptoms of lactose intolerance appear. It is important for people to understand that not only milk, but *any* milk product, can cause the symptoms of lactose intolerance in someone with diminished levels of lactase.

The incidence of lactose intolerance is very high among certain ethnic groups. For example, up to 75 percent of all African-Americans, Jewish, Native Americans, and Mexican-Americans are lactose intolerant. It is less common among northern Europeans, but up to 90 percent of Asian-Americans are lactose intolerant. Approximately, 75 percent of the world population is lactose intolerant.

Most patients with lactose intolerance have the hereditary delayed onset type. It can, however, be associated with other gastrointestinal disorders such as infectious gastroenteritis, inflammatory bowel disease (such as Crohn's disease), or celiac sprue. In these diseases, injury to the lining of the small intestine can decrease the amount of lactase that is produced. Often, patients with Crohn's disease or celiac sprue will have an unmasking of latent lactose intolerance or an increase in their known lactose intolerance when their primary gastrointestinal disorder flares.

Lactose intolerance must be differentiated from other gastrointestinal disorders. The symptoms of lactose intolerance are similar to those of the irritable bowel syndrome which can cause abdominal cramps, nausea, gas, and diarrhea. More serious diseases such as celiac sprue, inflammatory bowel disease (Crohn's disease and ulcerative colitis), or various infections need to be excluded. Because lactose intolerance and irritable bowel syndrome are very common, they can often coexist. Both disorders may have to be treated to get full resolution of symptoms.

Lactose intolerance can often be diagnosed clinically. The association of milk products along with the typical symptoms often gives the diagnosis. Avoiding milk products for several days, with clearing of the symptoms, makes the diagnosis. If the diagnosis is unclear, several tests can be done. The lactose intolerance test measures blood sugar (glucose) after the ingestion of a lactose-containing liquid. Lactase breaks down the lactose into glucose and galactose. If the blood sugar level does not rise appropriately, then lactose intolerance is present. Other less commonly used tests include the hydrogen breath test and stool acidity (ph) test. The latter test is used in young children.

The treatment of lactose intolerance is lactose restriction. Remember that it is the sugar, not the fat, in milk that is the problem. Low fat milk may be good for your cholesterol, but it will not help lactose intolerance. Lactose-reduced milk which contains the additions of the enzyme lactase is helpful. Lactase tablets, capsules, and the liquid can be added to the milk product or ingested just prior to the milk product. This will often prevent the symptoms of lactose intolerance. One must be sure to take enough of these tablets (often 3 or 4 tablets) to prevent the symptoms. This will vary with an individual's sensitivity to lactose.

Lactose intolerance is a very common disorder. It is usually not serious unless associated with other disorders such as Crohn's disease or celiac sprue. Depending on the degree of lactose intolerance, however, the symptoms can be quite disturbing. The use of lactase products and better understanding of this disorder have greatly improved its management.

A dietary guide of this type offers tasty, attractive lactose-free recipes. It is also a guide to commercially available food and suggestions in ways to help improve the management of lactose intolerance. This can be an important assistance for the lactose-impaired person, so that he or she, too, can enjoy healthy and happy eating.

FRANK R. MALKIN, M.D., F.A.C.G.
Metro West Medical Center
Natick, Massachusetts

PREFACE AND ACKNOWLEDGMENTS

This book is the result of a personal need. Several years ago, I became lactose intolerant—one of approximately 50 million Americans who cannot digest dairy products.

Although I am neither a nutritionist nor a physician, I am the author of another special-needs cookbook, *So What If You Can't Chew, Eat Hearty!* It was specifically designed as a guide and recipe book for the orally compromised person.

Because I saw the need for a similar guide and cookbook for the person who is lactose intolerant, I took up the challenge to write this book, *How To Tolerate Lactose Intolerance.*

I researched my files for recipes that could be converted or adjusted to satisfy the nutritional needs of a person who is lactose intolerant, and to provide excellent and tasty meals for the entire family.

My research also took me to Medical libraries for the latest literature on lactose intolerance and nutrition, to the pharmaceutical industry and to "fast food" corporations, airlines, supermarkets, health food stores, and restaurants. This helped to provide me with a comprehensive study of lactose intolerance, and knowledge of how to eat well and happily without dairy products.

A cookbook and guide of this kind cannot be written without help, advice, and encouragement. Therefore, I am indebted to authors of other cookbooks and friends who readily shared their favorite recipes—only to have them redone by me.

My special thanks must go to:

Frank R. Malkin, M.D., F.A.C.G., Gastroenterologist, MetroWest Medical Centers, Framingham and Natick, Massachusetts

Judith H. Jerome, for the illustrations and cover design

Marilyn G. Nemarich, for typing the manuscript

Shirley Z. Rosenthal, for proofreading

Harriet J. Kei, for proofreading

Morton H. Goldberg, D.M.D., M.D., my husband, for his readily available help and advice in preparing this book.

CONTENTS

HOW TO TOLERATE LACTOSE INTOLERANCE

Chapter 1

WHAT IS LACTOSE INTOLERANCE?

"There are two elements in daily products that must be broken down by enzymes in the body in order to be digested: lactose and caesin. Lactose is broken down by the enzyme lactase and caesin is broken down by the enzyme rennin. By ages three or four, rennin is nonexistent in the human digestive tract and in all but a small number of people, so is lactase. Those individuals who cannot digest lactose are known as being lactose intolerant." [1]

Lactose Intolerance (LI) is not a rare occurrence. It is estimated that in the United States alone, there are 50 million people who are LI in some form that may be mild, moderate, or severe. The symptoms can range from mild gas pains and cramps to severe diarrhea.

"Theories have been offered to suggest why certain racial and ethnic groups have genetically-transmitted LI and to explain the high incidence in the African and Asian populations. One theory is that genetic selection gives some groups high intestinal levels of lactase and others low levels. A low incidence of lactose intolerance may have developed in groups that have a high abundance of milk in their diets because of its ready availability. Conversely, lactose intolerance probably developed in a higher incidence in ethnic groups where milk products are rarely included in the adult diet. It has also been suggested that after weaning, the loss of lactase occures with maturation and is the normal condition for man." [2]

Chapter 2

BEWARE AND BE AWARE OF HIDDEN LACTOSE

Reading labels on the food products you consume is the first line of defense in avoiding products that contain lactose. Don't be fooled into thinking that if it is not in the dairy section, it does not contain lactose.

Beware of ingredients that have words like, whey, dry milk, solids, milk by-products, and curds. They most likely will contain lactose. Those ingredients can be found anywhere on the list on the package.

Be aware of convenience foods and food products we all commonly use which may contain even small amounts of lactose:

Sandwich breads
Cereals, high protein and instant cereals
Pancakes and waffles
Certain margarines
Instant breakfast mixes
Some instant coffees
Cream cordials and liqueurs
Cocoa mixes
Breaded frozen foods
Luncheon meats and hotdogs
French-fries and instant mashed potatoes
Cream-style soups
Creamy salad dressings and dips
Mayonnaise
Creamed vegetables
Sherbet
"Store bought" cookies
Suger substitutes

Some nondairy/whipped creamers
Commercially prepared gravy
Canned and frozen fruit
Chewing gum
Candies
Caramels, fudge, and milk chocolate
Packaged cake and cookies mixes
Commercial pie crusts and pie fillings
Puddings and custards

Not all of these products have lactose, so reading the ingredient list is important.

PAREVE

To be absolutely, positively sure that the product does not contain lactose, look for the work "pareve" (pronounced parve) on the product package. It is a Yiddish word meaning that is was prepared without either meat or dairy product in accordance with Kosher laws. Look for this label U Pareve. The "U" means Kosher. However, not all Kosher foods are Pareve.

Chapter 3

LACTOSE IN SOME COMMONLY-USED DRUGS

Lactose is often used as a filler and binder in many capsules and tablets. This includes prescription drugs as well as over-the-counter medications, including some vitamins. Many commercial drug companies now list "lactose free" on their labels. It is always wise to consult your pharmacist for more information (see chart).

Below are some commonly used drugs in which lactose is used as a filler in its preparation. Remember that there is a risk/benefit ratio. Do the risks out weigh the benefits, or vise versa? In other words, do you need the drug enough to risk the side effects of using a drug with a lactose filler*

Drug	Type	Inactive Filler	Company
Darvon Darvolcet	analgesic	lactose	Eli Lilly
Pen Veek	antibiotic (penicillin)	lactose Liquid-lactose-free	Wyeth Ayerst
Inderal	beta blocker anti-hyprtension	lactose	Wyeth Ayerst
Lopressor	beta blocker	lactose	Geigy
Ortho-novum	birth control	lactose	Ortho
Premarin	estrogen	lactose	Wyeth Ayerst
Immodium A-D	anti diarrheal	lactose	McNeil
Elavil	mood elevator	lactose	Stuart
Ansaid	nonsteroidal antiiinflamatory	lactose	Upjohn

* List compiled from *Physicians' Desk Reference, 1995.*

Chapter 4

A WORD ABOUT COMMERCIAL SUPPLEMENTS

Whether or not your aim is to gain weight or lose weight, there is a liquid supplement for you, and being LI, you must be aware of the ingredients and how they may affect you.

Commerically-prepared, high protein, dietary supplements are canned, balanced meals in liquid and powdered forms, and each contains 240 to 250 calories per serving. They will probably be suggested for use by your physician or dentist to boost your caloric intake. However, they should not be used as a substitute for balanced meals. The canned liquid supplements contain *no lactose.* If the powder form is used, substitute soy milk, enriched rice milk, or Lactaid® milk for the dairy milk usually required for mixing with the powder. These are sold in grocery stores and drug stores (food stamps allowed) under the trade names of Ensure®, Sustacal® and others.

If you are among the millions of people who desire to be svelte and want to lose weight by going on a liquid diet like Slim Fast®, or Ultra Slim Fast®, be aware that the products *do contain lactose* as they are commercially mixed with dairy products.

Chapter 5

LACTOSE CONTENT OF DAIRY FOODS

Food	Portion	Lactose (gm)
Cheeses		
American, processed	1 ounce	2.5
cheddar	1 ounce	0.4
cottage, low-fat	4 ounces	3.0
cream	1 ounce	0.8
feta	1 ounce	1.2
hard	1 ounce	0 to 3.0
Muenster	1 ounce	0.3
soft	4 ounces	3 to 6
Cream (whipping, heavy, half and half)	1 Tbs.	0.4 to 0.6
Ice Cream	1 cup	9 to 10
Milk		
goat's milk	8 ounces	10.9
skim	8 ounces	11.9
whole	8 ounces	11.4
Yogurt		
regular	8 ounces	10.6
skim (added nonfat dry milk)	8 ounces	17.4

Chapter 6

THE FOOD PYRAMID

The U.S. Department of Agriculture has revamped the four basic food groups we all know so well. The pyramid concept, adopted in 1992, recommends daily servings of those food groups: breads and cereals; fruits and vegetables; dairy and meats; and fats, oils, and sweets. At a glance, you can view which food groups contribute more to a good daily diet. About two-thirds up on the pyramid are dairy products (milk, cheese, and yogurt) of which two or three servings are recommended daily.

If you are LI, do not despair. The lactose-free milks that are available (enriched rice, soy, prepared lactose-free products) give a person the same nutrients necessary to maintain a balanced diet that is urged by the U.S.D.A. See pyramid on next page.

THE FOOD GUIDE PYRAMID
A Guide to Daily Food Choices

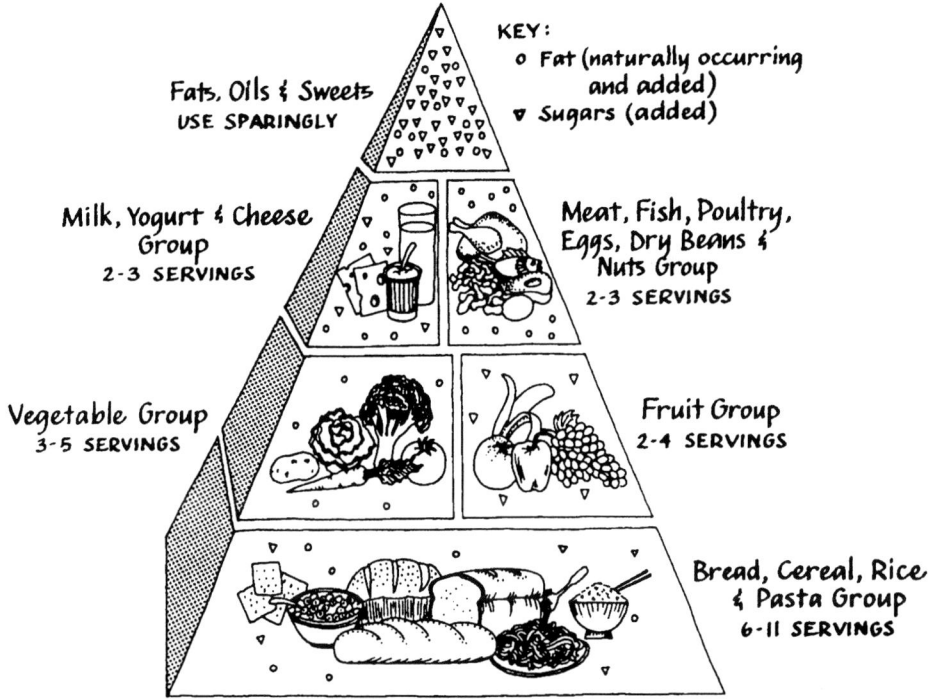

KEY:
o Fat (naturally occurring and added)
▽ Sugars (added)

Fats, Oils & Sweets
USE SPARINGLY

Milk, Yogurt & Cheese
Group
2-3 SERVINGS

Meat, Fish, Poultry,
Eggs, Dry Beans &
Nuts Group
2-3 SERVINGS

Vegetable Group
3-5 SERVINGS

Fruit Group
2-4 SERVINGS

Bread, Cereal, Rice
& Pasta Group
6-11 SERVINGS

CREDIT: U.S. Department of Agriculture, Human Nutrition Information Service

Chapter 7

OSTEOPOROSIS AND CALCIUM

The need for calcium for good health cannot be underestimated. If you are LI, you may be denied a major source of calcium-rich dairy products. The lack of calcium can contribute to the loss of bone called osteoporosis. It can occur in both men and women, but women are at a higher risk because of diminished estrogen in their bodies. One out of three women suffers from this bone disease after menopause.

During the teen years, there is mass bone formation. A diet low in calcium can limit bone formation at this time. The greater the bone mass obtained early in life, the larger the reserve will be in later years.

Although calcium is essential for maintaining the health of your bones and teeth, it also helps to contract muscles, clot blood, and aids the nerves to carry messages.

The two methods in which your body obtains calcium are from diet and from your bones. Because calcium in not produced within your body, it must come from your diet, which spares and protects the calcium in your bones. If the calcium level is too low for your bodily needs, it will be drawn from the bones, thereby weakening them and the skeletal structure.

It is a known fact that more women than men suffer from osteoporosis. However, studies show that as men age, their incidence of hip fractures also increases. The recommended dietary allowance (RDA) for teens is 1,200 milligrams of calcium a day. For women, ages 25 to 40, it is 1,000 milligrams and for over 40 years of age, 1,500 milligrams. Calcium needs rise with pregnancy, as the mother must meet her needs as well as those of the growing fetus. The RDA is 1,200 milligrams daily for the nursing mother (see the chart on page 16).

Being LI does not represent a problem in meeting those needs because enriched rice milk, soy milk, and lactose-reduced milk contain the same level of calcium found in dairy milk. Remember, too, that calcium-fortified bread and orange juice can help meet your dietary needs.

One should also get plenty of sun exposure because sunlight is necessary for the body to produce vitamin D, which helps the body absorb and maintain normal levels of calcium. As a caution, however, some studies suggest that using sunscreen can lower blood levels of vitamin D. It is suggested that if a person wants to obtain the required amount of vitamin D, he or she should expose his or her face, arms, and hands to about 10 to 15 minutes on early morning or late afternoon sun, two or three times a week. Sunscreen with a SPF of at least #15 should be used the rest of the time in order to reduce the risk of skin cancer. For the LI person, dietary sources of vitamin D are oily fish such as salmon, herring, and sardines; cod liver oil; and egg yolks. No more than 400 International Units should be taken daily. If you feel that you are not meeting these requirements, consult your physician about dietary supplements.

As a word of caution: it would be wise to reduce your intake of caffeine and alcohol as they can interfere with the body's absorption of calcium from food.

National Institute of Health Chart

(Based on milligrams of calcium requirement per day)

Birth-6 months	400
Age 1-10 years	600
Age 11-24 years	800-1,200
Women under age 24 (pregnant and lactating)	1,200-1,500
Women over age 24 (pregnant and lactating)	1,200

Women 25-49 years (pre-menopausal)	1,000
Women 50-64 (post menopausal and taking estrogen)	1,000
Women 50-64 years (post menopausal and not taking estrogen)	1,500
Men (25-64 years)	1,500
Women and Men over 65	1,500

Other Sources of Calcium

Fortified, or enriched, Rice Dream Nondairy Beverage®	1 cup	300 mg
Broccoli	1/2 cup	36 mg
Kale (cooked)	3 oz	61 mg
Pinto beans	1/2 cup	75 mg
Sardines	2 oz	134 mg
Tofu	3 oz	89 mg

Drugs That Cause Calcium Loss

Aluminum-containing antacids
Dilantin
Heparin
Lithium
Phenobarbital

Phenothiazine derivatives
Tetracycline
Thyroid hormone

Please consult your physician if you are taking any of these medications. He or she may advise you on an appropriate calcium supplement.

Fast
Foods

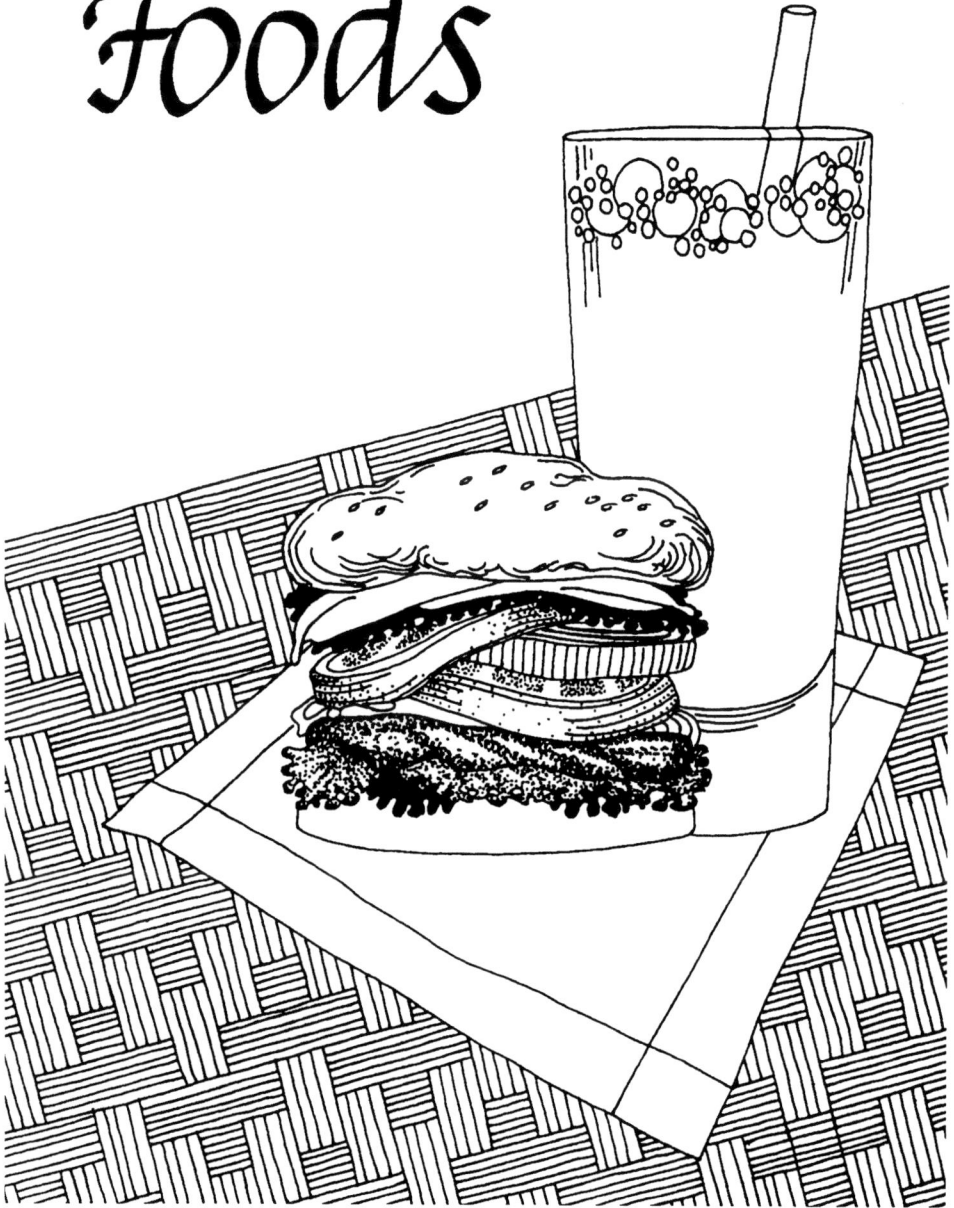

Chapter 8

FAST FOODS CAN STILL BE FUN

Going to a popular fast food restaurant has become an international pastime enjoyed by millions. If you are Lactose intolerant, you can still eat with gusto–just be aware that your choices should fit your LI sensitivity.

McDonalds

The following items contain MILK and LACTOSE:

birthday cakes

biscuits

breakfast burrito: cheese tortilla (may contain whey)

butter

cheddar melt sauce

cheese

chicken fajitas tortilla (may contain whey)

Chicken McNuggets

McChicken patty

cookies–chocolaty chip

croutons

Danish pastry

eggs (may be cooked in butter)

fish fillet

half & half creamer

hotcakes

hot chocolate

lowfat frozen yogurt

lowfat milk shakes (all)

margarine pats

milk

muffins: fat-free, apple bran, fat-free blueberry

pies (all)

salads (shredded cheese), chef salad

salad dressings: bleu cheese, ranch, 1000 island

soups: broccoli cheese, cream of potato, New England clam
        chowder

sundae toppings: caramel and fudge

whipped cream

This looks like a long list, but there is still a huge variety from which to choose.

Subway

Subway® Sandwich Shops urges customers with dietary restrictions to inquire at each individual store about specific dietary contents of the food products, as they may vary from region to region.

The following food items *do not* contain milk products:

turkey bologna	turkey salami
turkey ham	steak
pepperoni	bacon
roast beef	marinara sauce
roasted chicken breast fillet	tuna
Subway® seafood and crab	vegetables–lettuce, tomatoes, olives, onions, pickles, green peppers, jalapeno pepper slices,
all condiments	thousand island dressing

fat-free italian dressing   light mayonnaise
                              dressing

Be aware that all of the varieties of Subway cookies contain some form of milk product as milk lactose or whey.

Wendy's

Products containing Lactose, Casein, Whey, and Curds:

kaiser and sandwich buns	American cheese slices
blue cheese	Italian caesar dressing
Hidden Valley® Ranch dressing	reduced fat ranch dressing
taco salad	alfredo sauce
cheese sauce	macaroni and cheese
roma parmesan blend	sour cream topping
bacon and cheese potato	broccoli and cheese potato
cheese potato	sour cream and chives potato
chili and cheese potato	whipped margarine
cheddar cheese, shredded	crispy chicken nuggets
Frosty® dairy dessert	chocolate chip cookie
hot chocolate	cheddar chips (salad)
croutons	cottage cheese
vanilla pudding	chocolate pudding

KFC
Kentucky Fried Chicken

The following menu items do not contain lactose:

hot wings	honey barbecue wings
Colonel's Rotessorie Gold	potato wedges

cole slaw   potato salad
corn-on-the cob   barbecued baked beans
chicken sandwich   apple pie slices

Boston Market

The following menu items contain milk and lactose:

brownies   home style mashed potatoes
butternut squash   Mediterranean pasta salad
buttered corn   macaroni & cheese
caesar salad   oatmeal raisin cookie
chicken pot pie   savory rice pilaf
caesar salad with   old fashioned chicken soup
  chicken
chocolate chip cookies   spicy smashed potatoes
corn bread   stuffing
creamed spinach   tortellini salad
garlic & dill new   vegetable pot pie
  potatoes
gravy   ham
turkey   meatloaf

The following are recommended alternatives:

BBQ baked beans   fresh fruit salad
chicken breast   fresh steamed vegetables
  sandwich
chunky chicken   garden fresh cole slaw
  salad
chunky chicken   honey dijon dressing
  salad sandwich
cinnamon apples   potato salad
cranberry walnut   rotisserie chicken
  relish
cucumber salad   zucchini marinara

Taco Bell

The following menu items contain milk or dry milk solids:

whole milk	soft tacos
all of the cheeses	caramel rolls
flour tortillas	sour cream
burritos	guacamole

One should choose other menu items and ask the manager for particular suggestions.

Dunkin Donuts

Unfortunately, all doughnut products are made with milk and milk solids. This is true of most all commercial store-variety doughnut products as well.

Dining Out

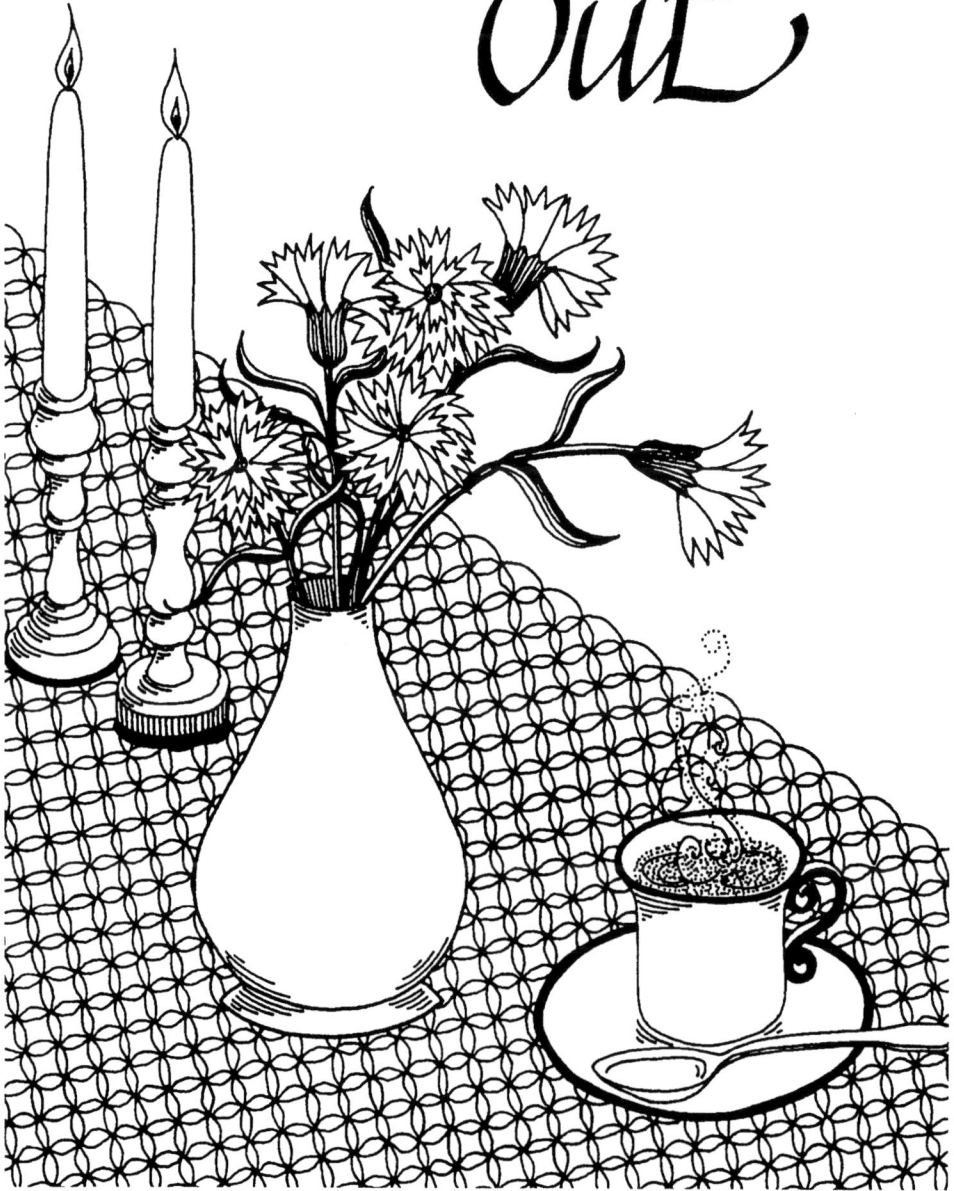

Chapter 9

DINING OUT

Dining out at a restaurant can be either a pleasure or a challenge for a person who is lactose intolerant. The menus are replete with enticing and wonderful sounding dishes–but where do you begin?

1. Read the menu thoroughly.

2. Pick out the dishes that appeal to your appetite and your senses.

3. If you are at all unsure if there are any dairy products used in the preparation of a particular dish, ask the server to ask the chef. Don't be shy. Most servers will be happy to comply. They, themselves, may know how the dish is prepared.

4. With this information at hand, place your order. If the dish comes with a sauce, it is always wise to have it served on the side so that you may use it at *your* discretion. If an error is made, have them correct it.

Salads

Stay away from "creamy" anything. Italian dressings are usually prepared with Parmesan or Romano cheese, unless your server tells you otherwise. French dressings are usually okay, but the ranch type is a definate "no-no". To be really safe, stick to oil and vinegar.

Soups

Again, avoid anything with "cream of" in the name of soup. Some Italian soups, like minestrone, can be prepared with cheeses. Ask your server. If the cheese is added later, tell the waiter to "hold" yours. Another popular gourmet soup is French onion soup which is both very rich and very delicious. However, for the LI person, it is the wrong soup to eat. In its preparation, a large buttered crouton is placed at the bottom of the bowl with a baked layer of cheese on top. If you love onions, perhaps the chef can prepare a bowl for you without the crouton or the cheese. The onion broth can be wonderful. It doesn't hurt to ask.

Appetizers

Many appetizers are prepared with cheeses of one sort or another. Some restaurants offer shrimp, chopped liver or a small pasta-like dish (without cheese). Similar offerings can be considered acceptable to eat. Remember, ask you server.

Entrees

Steaks and chops are always a safe bet. Chicken prepared without a dairy-based sauce, stuffing, or breading can be a good choice. Fish or seafood are also good choices, if prepared without stuffing or breading. Watch the toppings too. Inform the server that you cannot have *any* dairy products and ask if the chef can prepare your selection with lemon juice or wine. NO butter, please.

If you are a vegetarian, or just a pasta lover, consider a marinara sauce. Meatballs are often prepared with bread crumbs that contain cheese. More hidden lactose!

Ethnic Restaurants

Ethnic restaurants can be tricky unless you know the language or are familiar with the foods. If you are not, be sure to ask the server or the chef for help in your selection. If the server does not understand your request, you may be on your own. Sometimes, descriptions of menu selections are provided. One may also enlist the aid of other diners. As a friendly gesture, they may help.

Dining Out in Someone's Home

If you have been invited to someone's home for a dinner party, it may be a good idea to let the host know in advance that you are lactose intolerant. This information can avoid embarrassment for you and your host. This gives them a chance to include food that you can eat too. They can add a fresh fruit cocktail or extra vegetables, without butter, that would be a good complement to their menu. Remember, there is usually bread to assuage your hunger.

Desserts

Whether you are in a restaurant or in someone's home, dessert can be a problem. If it seems that the best desserts are made with all the things you cannot eat, you are probably right!

If fruit is offered anywhere on the menu, order it. If a thoughtful host has considered a sorbet, enjoy it. You may have to bite the bullet and have only coffee or tea. However, do not hesitate to ask if something contains a dairy product (your stomach will thank you).

Take Lactaid® or other supplement tablets with you at all times. These products contains the enzyme lactase that makes dairy food more digestible. Experience will help you find the proper amount for you. Be sure to have an ample supply. You never know when you will need them and they may help. Meanwhile, Mangia! Bon Appetit!

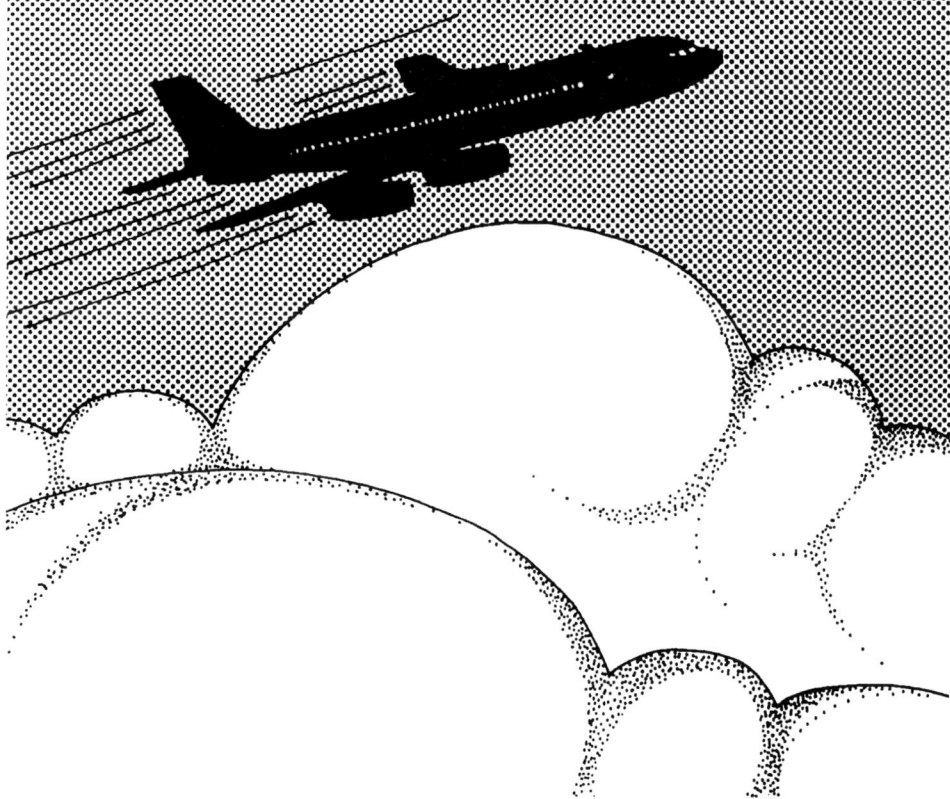

Airline
Foods

Chapter 10

AIRLINE MEALS

All the major airlines offer meals that are compatible with a lactose intolerant diet. However, meals are not served on flights less than 2 to 2 1/2 hours duration. In order to insure that you can have lactose-free meals, and therefore a more pleasant journey, here are some suggestions:

1. Inform your travel agent or airline representative that you want lactose-free meals. The choices can include:
   a. Vegetarian meals
   b. Fruit plates (even breakfast)
   c. Kosher meals (there is no guarantee whether this would be a meat or dairy meal. If it is a meat meal, all the courses will be "pareve" (no dairy products). Stress your preference strongly.
   d. Lacto-ovo meals (nondairy/no eggs)

2. Bring your own meal aboard the plane, especially if you know it will be a meal-less flight. Purchase a meal in one of the airport's courtyard restaurants before boarding the aircraft. You can get the beverage of you choice on board.

3. Bring something to eat from home. My husband and I always take a couple of split bagels, already peanut buttered in a plastic bag. They are tasty, nutritious, neat to eat, and on short flights, very satisfying. With juice and coffee, you can enjoy breakfast or lunch.

So, travelers, don't despair, plan ahead for your trip and life on a plane can be more than a tiny bag of peanuts.

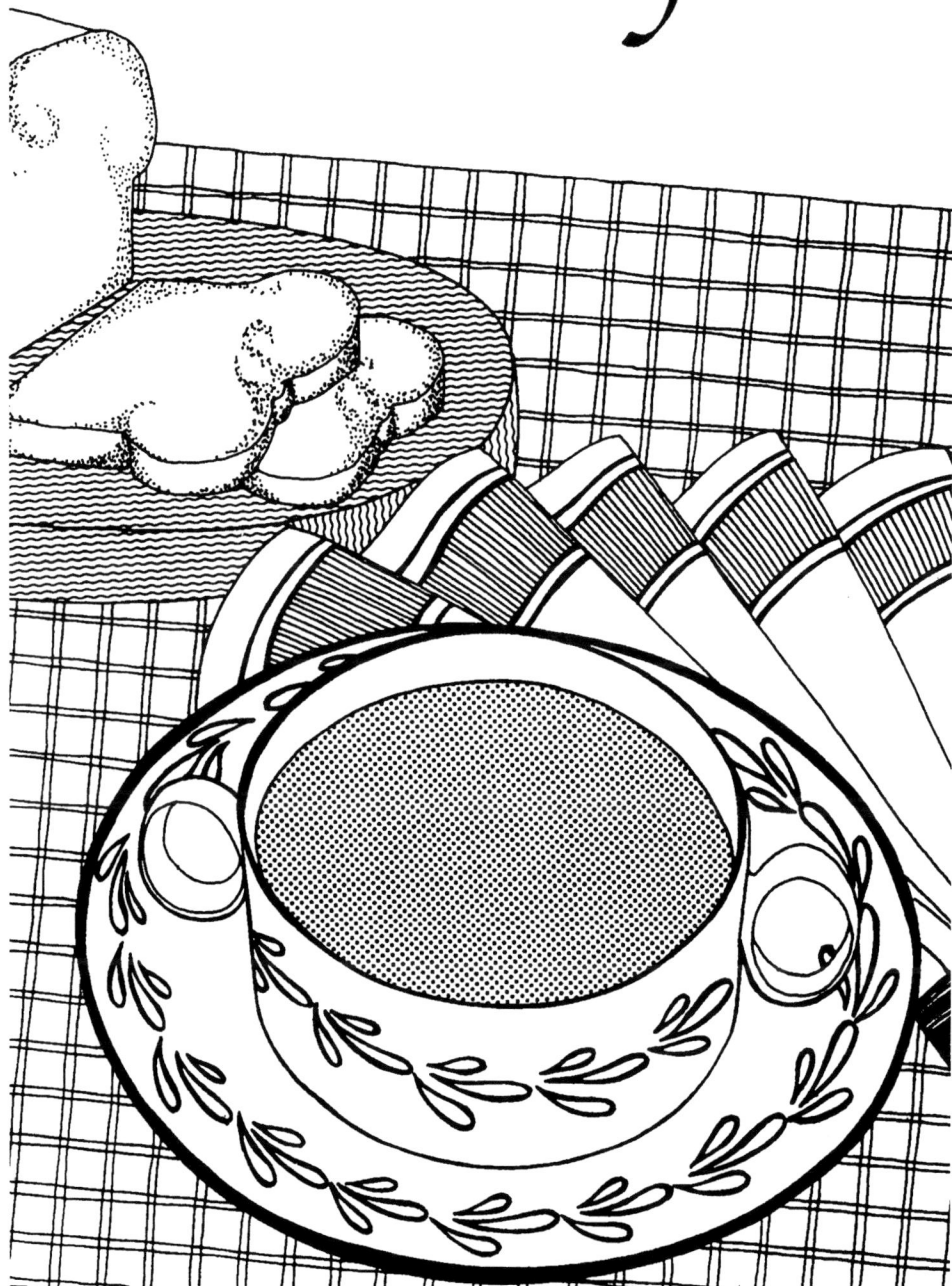

Soups

Chapter 11

SOUPS

"CREAM" SOUP
Let's Pretend

1 medium onion, cut up
2 medium celery stalks, cut up
2 cloves pressed garlic
4 cups vegetables cut up (broccoli, asparagus,
   carrots, squash, potatoes–your choice!)
5 cups water
2 bullion cubes (chicken or vegetable)
2 tablespoons olive oil

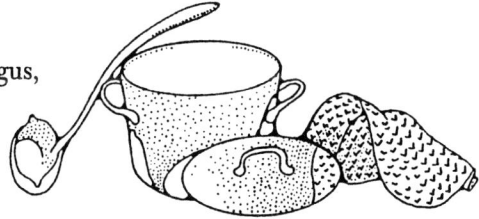

Heat oil, onion, celery, and garlic in a large soup pot. Sauté for 10 minutes on low heat. Stir often. Add cut up vegetables and cubes. Cook on
low heat until vegetables are very tender (10-15 minutes). Cool in
refrigerator for 4 hours or overnight. Put through the blender until
smooth. Season with pepper or curry to taste. Serve with sprinkled
parsley or chives.

CARROT SOUP*
A Sunny Surprise

1 1/2 pounds carrots, peeled and sliced
4 cups water
1 teaspoon salt
1/2 small onion
10 1/2 ounces soft silken tofu (regular or low fat)
1 teaspoon dried dill
pepper

Boil carrots and onion in water until tender. Place carrots and onion in a blender. Add tofu and dill. Puree. Return puree to cooking water. Mix well. Serve hot or cold.

* See Chapter 14.

"CREAM" OF TOMATO-BASIL SOUP
Serve this hot in the winter—cold in the summer

1 28-ounce can crushed tomatoes
1/3 cup Farm Fresh* Fat-Free Creamer
1 tablespoon flour
1/2 tsp. dried basil
1 tablespoon lemon juice
1/2 teaspoon salt (or to taste)
1/4 teaspoon pepper

Put the contents of the can of tomatoes in a blender and puree. Combine the creamer and the flour until smooth. Into the blender container, add this mixture and the remaining ingredients. Mix well in the blender. Pour into a sauce pan and bring to a boil. Lower the heat and cook for 5 minutes. Serve hot or refrigerate the soup for 6 hours until well chilled. Garnish with chives.

PUMPKIN PECAN BISQUE
An Autumn Delight

2 tablespoon margarine
1 cup chopped onion
1 garlic clove (minced)
14-1/2 ounce can chicken broth (1 3/4 cups)
16 ounce can solid pack pumpkin (1 3/4 cup)
1 1/4 cups water
1 teaspoon brown sugar
1/2 teaspoon dried thyme
1/2 teaspoon cumin
1/4 teaspoon salt
1 cup pecan pieces, toasted
1 1/2 cups Farm Rich® Non-Dairy Creamer

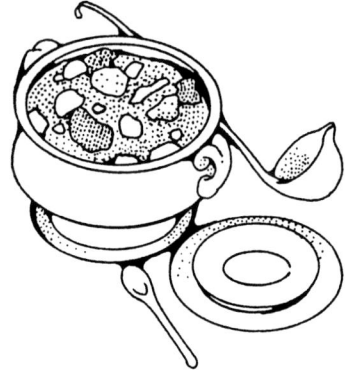

In a large saucepan, melt margarine (no lactose, please). Add onion and saute 6 minutes over medium heat. Add garlic and saute until slightly browned. Add chicken broth, pumpkin, water, sugar, thyme, cumin, and salt. Bring to simmer over medium heat, reduce heat and cook 10 minutes, stirring frequently. Remove from heat and add pecan pieces. Cool thoroughly. Puree in a blender or food processor. Stir in the Farm Rich until in incorporated.

Hint: to toast pecans, preheat oven to 350 degrees F. Spread pecans in shallow pan and bake until golden brown (about 5 to 10 minutes).

CORN CHOWDER
Down East Treat

2 tablespoon margarine
1/2 cup chopped onion
2 tablespoons flour
2 cups water
1 cup small cubed potatoes
1 cup creamed style corn
1 1/2 cups Farm Fresh Creamer (Skim or original)
salt and pepper to taste

Saute onion in margarine. Add flour and make a roux. Add water, potatoes, and corn. Cook until tender. Add milk, salt, and pepper. Heat and serve.

QUICK "CHEESE" SOUP
Easy too!

1 cup sliced celery
1 cup chopped onion
2 tablespoons margarine
2/3 cup flour
4 cups water or chicken broth or 6 low salt
   chicken bullion cubes
1 cup potatoes (canned is OK)
1 package frozen vegetable combination
3 cups Rice Dream® Rice Milk.
2 1/2 cups Smart Beat® no-lactose cheese alternative
1/4 teaspoon pepper

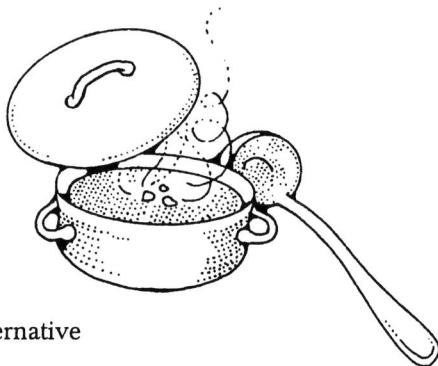

Cook celery and onion in margarine until tender. Stir in flour until smooth. Add water or broth or bullion. Add dash pepper. Bring to a boil. Add milk and cheese. Cook until cheese melts.

AVOCADO SOUP
California, here I come!

1/2 large avocado, peeled, seeded, and sliced
3/4 cup chicken broth
1/2 minced garlic clove
dash Tabasco® sauce
2 ice cubes
1/4 cup rice milk

Place all ingredients except rice milk into blender. Blend for 15 seconds. Wit motor running on low speed, remove cover and slowly add ice cubes and rice milk. On high speed, blend 30 seconds. Serve hot or cold.

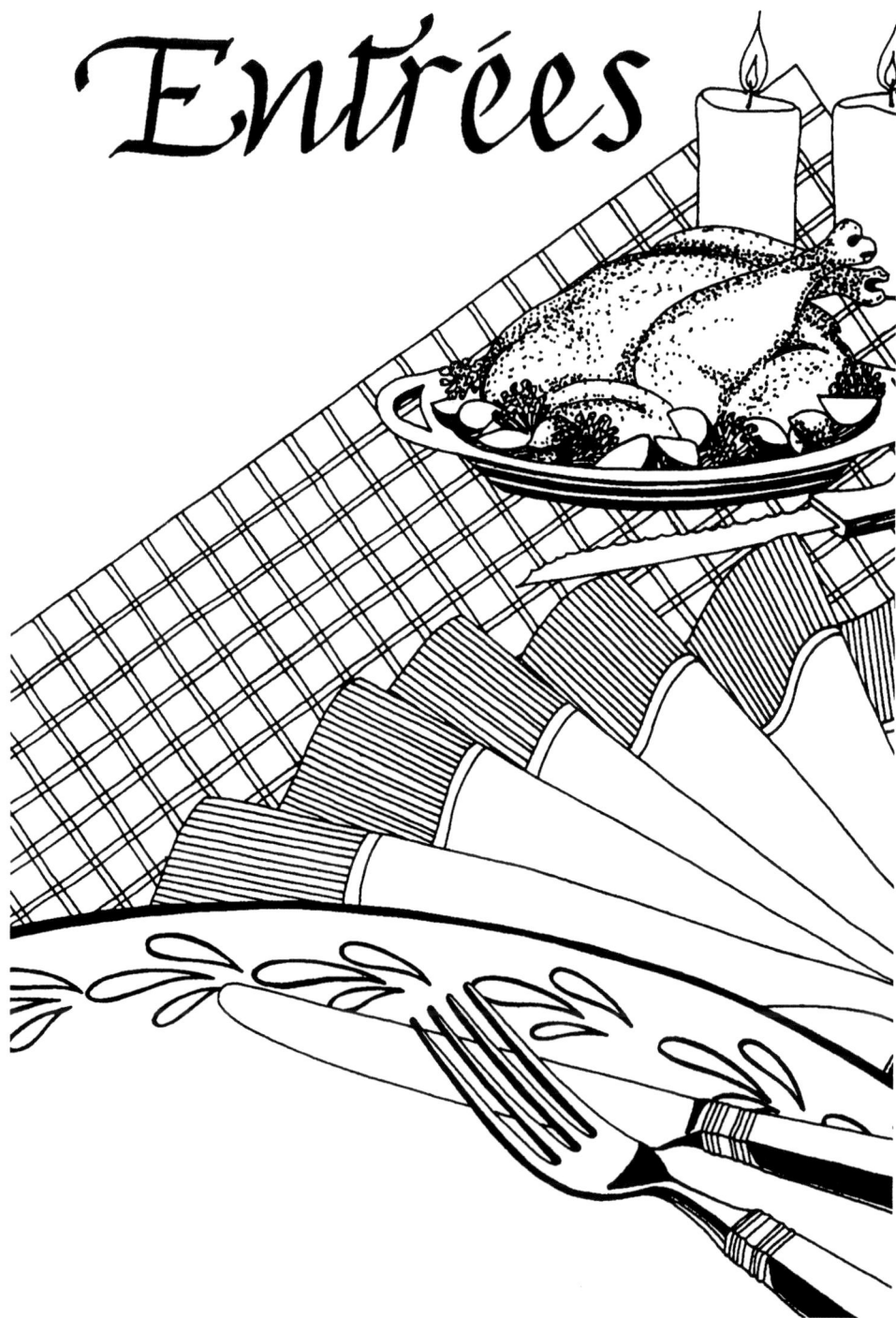

Entrées

Chapter 12

ENTREES

SHIRLEY'S R'S POACHED FISH
It's super with sauce

Fill frying pan 1/2 inch deep with Lactaid® 100% Lactose Reduced milk, and heat to just below boiling point. Add 1 pound of fish. Reduce heat and cook gently until the fish flakes when fork tested. Lift fish out gently, and serve with egg sauce.

Egg Sauce
1/3 cup margarine (check for milk product)
3 tablespoons flour
1 1/2 cups hot water
1/2 teaspoon salt
dash pepper
2 egg yolks, beaten
1 teaspoon lemon juice

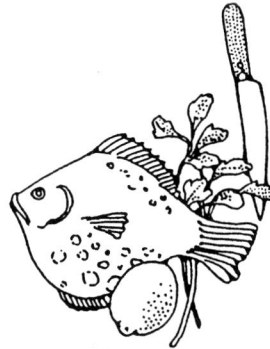

Mix first four ingredients together (using a wisk helps). Gradually add the hot water. Slowly add beaten egg yolks and lemon juice. Serve over hot fish.

FELSON'S FISH FILLET
Serve this with a flair!

1 tablespoon margarine (Caution! Check the label.)
1/4 cup water
1/8 teaspoon powdered instant chicken bouillon
1 filet of sole or other similar fish
dash of onion powder
dash celery powder or pinch of celery seed
dash of dill

In a large saucepan, melt margarine in water, add spices and fish. Cover and simmer 10 minutes or until fish flakes.

SALMON SOUFFLE
Easy and Elegant

1 pound of red sockeyed salmon
3 tablespoons flour
1/8 teaspoon pepper
1 cup Lactaid® 100% lactose reduced milk
  or Enriched Rice Dream vanilla milk
2 tablespoons lemon juice
1 tablespoon worcestershire sauce
1 tablespoon Tabasco sauce
3 egg yolks
3 egg whites

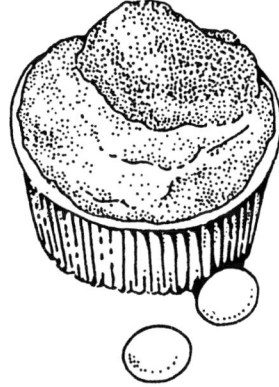

Place all ingredients in blender container and blend on high for 25 seconds. Pour into saucepan and cook over low heat until thickened. Stir frequently. Fold in 3 stiffly beaten egg whites. Transfer to a 1 1/2 quart souffle dish or one with higher sides. Bake in preheated 375 degree oven for 30 minutes or until it rises and lightly browns.

NEPTUNE CASSEROLE
A Deep Sea Delight

1–6 or 7 ounce can tunafish, water packed
8 ounce cooked sea shell shaped pasta
1 can Rokeach® brand barley and mushroom soup
3/4 can water (or Rice Dream rice milk)
1 tablespoon onion flakes
1/2 teaspoon garlic powder
dash chili powder (or to taste)
1 box frozen peas

Combine soup with either water or rice milk until smooth. Add flaked tuna and remaining ingredients. Place in a greased casserole and top with crushed chips. Cover with foil and bake in a 350 degree oven for 20 minutes. Uncover and continue baking for 10 minutes. Serves 4 to 6.

*Pronounced Ro-kay-ach. This soup product is dairy-free and "pareve" and can be found in the kosher food section of the supermarket.

5

SALMON PUFFS
Easy all-time favorite

2 slices white bread
1/8 teaspoon salt
1/4 teaspoon mustard
1/2 teaspoon minced onion
1/2 cup Farm Fresh Fat Free Creamer
1–3 1/2 ounce can salmon

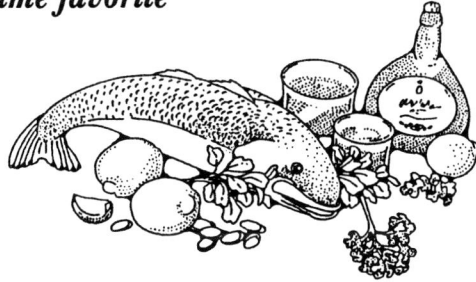

Into a blender container, place all ingredients along with the bread torn into small pieces. Blend for 20 seconds or until smooth. Don't debone salmon because bones are very soft, blend easily, and the extra calcium from the bones is a plus. Pour into a 1 1/2 quart baking dish and bake in a preheated 325 degree oven for 30-40 minutes until set and done. Serves four.

CRAB MOUSE
An awesome chip dip

1 envelope plain gelatin
1/2 cup hot chicken broth
2 egg yolks
2 1/2 ounces crab meat, flaked
dash or two Tabasco sauce
1/4 cup mayonnaise (read label)
1/2 stalk celery, cut into small pieces
1/4 teaspoon minced onion
3/4 teaspoon parsley
1/2 cup Farm Rich Non-Dairy Creamer
2 egg whites

Place gelatin and broth into container. Blend for 20 seconds. Add remaining ingredients, except creamer and egg whites. Blend for 15 seconds. Remove cover, and on low speed, add creamer. Turn crab mixture into stiffly beaten egg whites and fold in carefully. Chill until set.

Hint: For a gourmet touch, substitute 1/4 cup of white wine for 1/2 cup broth.

HOT QUOHOG STEW
It's Native American for clams

1–7 1/2 ounce can minced clams
1/2 teaspoon celery seed
dash of Tabasco
1/8 teaspoon tarragon
2 large potatoes peeled, cubed, boiled, and drained
3/4 cup Farm Fresh Original

Place all ingredients in a 1 1/2 quart casserole dish, cover and bake at 325 degrees for 25 to 30 minutes. Sprinkle with chives before serving.

TUNA POTATO PUFFS
A combination that's hard to beat

1–6 1/2 ounce can tuna fish (packed in water)
1 1/2 cups instant mashed potatoes
Rice Dream rice milk (enough to whip potatoes)
2 egg yolks beaten well or 1/4 cup of egg substitute
1/4 teaspoon salt
dash pepper
1 tablespoon minced onion
2 egg whites stiffly beaten

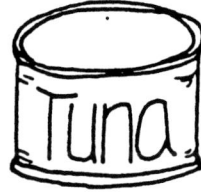

Drain and flake tuna. Mix with potatoes. Stir in egg yolks, salt, pepper, and onion. Blend 15 seconds. Fold in beaten egg whites. Spoon into six greased custard cups. Bake at 350 degrees for 30 minutes.

MILLY'S NO CHEESE LASAGNA
You don't even miss the mozzarella!

2 pounds ground beef, veal, turkey—or any
   combination mixed together to equal 2 pounds
3/4 cup chopped onion
2 tablespoons olive oil
1 can tomatoes
2–6 ounce cans tomato paste
2 cups water
1 tablespoon chopped parsley
2 teaspoons salt (or less)
1 teaspoon sugar
1 teaspoon garlic powder
1/2 teaspoon pepper
1/2 teaspoon oregano
8 ounce lasagna (1/2 package)

Brown meat and onion in oil. Add tomatoes (cut up or blend). Add rest of the ingredients, stirring occasionally about 30 minutes. Cook lasagna and drain. In 13 x 9 x 2 inch baking pan, spread 1 cup sauce, then alternate layers of lasagna and sauce, ending with sauce. Bake at 350 degrees for 40-50 minutes until lightly brown and bubbling. Allow to stand for 15 minutes. Cut into squares. Makes 8 servings.

OLD FASHIONED MASHED POTATOES
Smashed Spuds

Mash cooked potatoes (any variety). Add margarine to taste. Whip with enough Farm Fresh Non-dairy Creamer until the consistency pleases you. Add salt and pepper to taste. Onion powder can be used instead of salt. Top with dried parsley leaves.

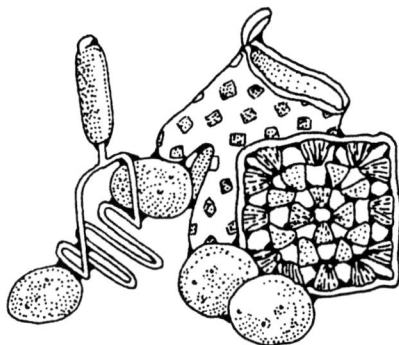

CURRIED CHICKEN DELUXE
Elegant

2 whole chicken breasts, boneless and skinless, cut into cubes
8 ounces mushrooms, sliced thin (can use canned)
1/3 cup chopped onion
1 tablespoon margarine
1 tablespoon canola oil
3 tablespoons flour
2 teaspoons instant chicken bullion
1 1/2 teaspoons curry powder (or to taste)
1 medium apple chopped fine
1/3 cup chopped parsley
1/2 cup Farm Rich Non-Dairy Creamer
3/4 cup water

Saute chicken, mushrooms, and onion in margarine and oil until chicken is lightly browned and completely cooked. Stir in flour and cook for 1 minute. Stir in bullion, curry, apple, and parsley. Gradually stir in Farm Rich and water, stirring constantly. Simmer, stirring for 4 to 5 minutes. Serve over rice or pasta. Makes 4 servings.

CHICKEN A LA KING
A Royal Dish

1 cup sliced mushrooms
3 tablespoons margarine
3 tablespoons flour
1/2 teaspoon salt
1/4 teaspoon pepper
2 cups Lactaid 100% lactose
 reduced milk or 1 cup each
 Farm Rich Original and water
2 cups chicken broth
2 1/2 cooked diced chicken
1 cup cooked peas
3 tablespoons pimento

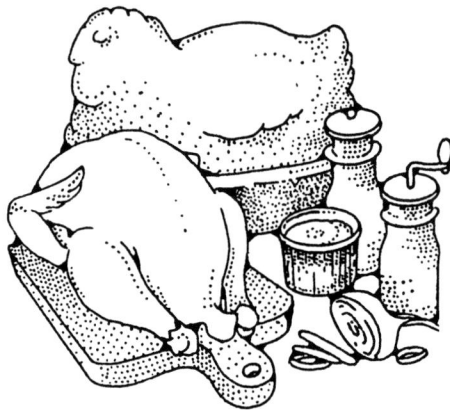

Sauté mushrooms in margarine. Slowly blend in flour, salt, and pepper. Stir in milk or chicken broth, peas, and pimento. Heat very well, Serve over rice or noodles.

TOFU RICOTTA*
Amazing!

1 1/2 pounds firm tofu, well mashed
1/4 cup lemon juice
1 1/2 tablespoon dried basil
1 tablespoon oregano
3/4 teaspoon salt
1/2 teaspoon garlic

Mash together all ingredients until the mixture has a grainy texture like ricotta. This may be stored in the refrigerator for up to 3 days. Tofu ricotta can be used in any dish that calls for dairy ricotta.

*See Chapter 14.

CARROT CASSEROLE
Sunshine on your plate

2 pounds carrots cooked and mashed
2 tablespoons margarine
1 onion, grated or instant equivalent
8 ounces Smart Beat cheese substitute
   (cheddar)
salt and pepper to taste
bread crumbs for topping

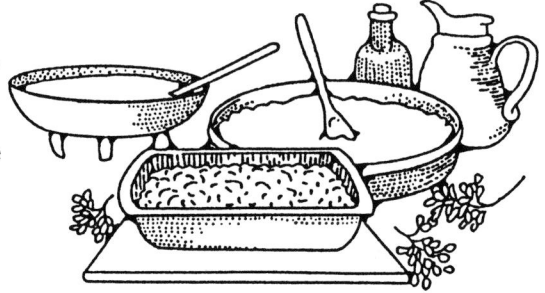

Combine carrots and onion. Place in a 1 1/2 quart casserole dish. Add "cheese" to cover carrots and onion. Sprinkle with bread crumbs. Dot with margarine. Bake at 350 degrees for 20 minutes until done or light brown.

MACARONI & "CHEESE"
Everyone's favorite

8 ounces macaroni
2 cups (8 oz.) Smart Beat nondairy American
  cheese flavored cheese substitute cut up into strips
1/4 teaspoon salt
1/4 teaspoon pepper
2 cups Lactaid milk (100% lactose reduced) or
  1 cup each Farm Rich Original and water
2 tablespoons margarine
paprika

Heat oven to 350 degrees. Place cooked macaroni in a 1 1/2 to 2 quart casserole dish that has been greased with margarine or sprayed with cooking oil. Cover with strips of Smart Beat cheese alternative, salt, and pepper. Dot with margarine. Pour Lactaid milk over the top and sprinkle with paprika. Cover and bake for 35 minutes. Uncover and bake again 14 minutes, or until top is browned.

"CHEESE" SOUFFLÉ
Elegant

1 cup diced Smart Beat no lactose cheese substitute
  (4 ounces cheddar or American)
2 tablespoons margarine
4 tablespoons flour
1/4 teaspoon dry mustard (optional)
1/2 teaspoon salt
5 egg yolks
1 cup hot Farm Fresh Fat-Free Non-dairy Creamer
5 egg whites, stiffly beaten

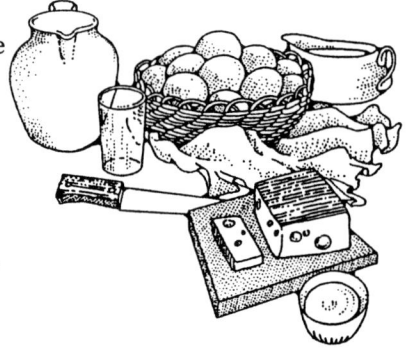

Put first seven ingredients into blender, and blend for 20 seconds. Pour mixture into a saucepan and cook over low heat until smooth and thick. Fold in egg whites and pour this mixture into a greased 1 1/2 quart soufflé dish. Bake at 375 degrees in preheated oven for 30 minutes. Serve immediately

*For egg soufflé, omit cheese.

AMERICAN CHOP SUEY
A kid's favorite supper!

12 ounces small pasta (elbows or small shells)
2 tablespoons vegetable oil
1/2 cup chopped celery
1/2 cup chopped green pepper
1 pound ground beef or turkey
1 can Rokeach® tomato soup
   (or other brand without dairy milk products)
salt and pepper to taste
2 cups shredded Smart Beat cheddar cheese
   flavored cheese substitute, divided

Preheat oven to 350 degrees. Boil pasta to al denté. Place in a large bowl. In a large skillet, sauté celery and green pepper in oil until tender. Drain off oil. Add ground meat to skillet and cook until there is no pink in the meat. Add mixture to the pasta. Stir in the tomato soup and 1/4 can water. Stir in 1 cup of cheese substitute. Place in a 2 quart casserole dish that has been coated with vegetable spray. Top with remaining cup of "cheese." Bake 30 minutes. Serve hot. (Crusty rolls or bread make this meal complete)

Hint: Rokeach food products can be found in the kosher food aisle of a large supermarket (pronounced Ro-kay-ach).

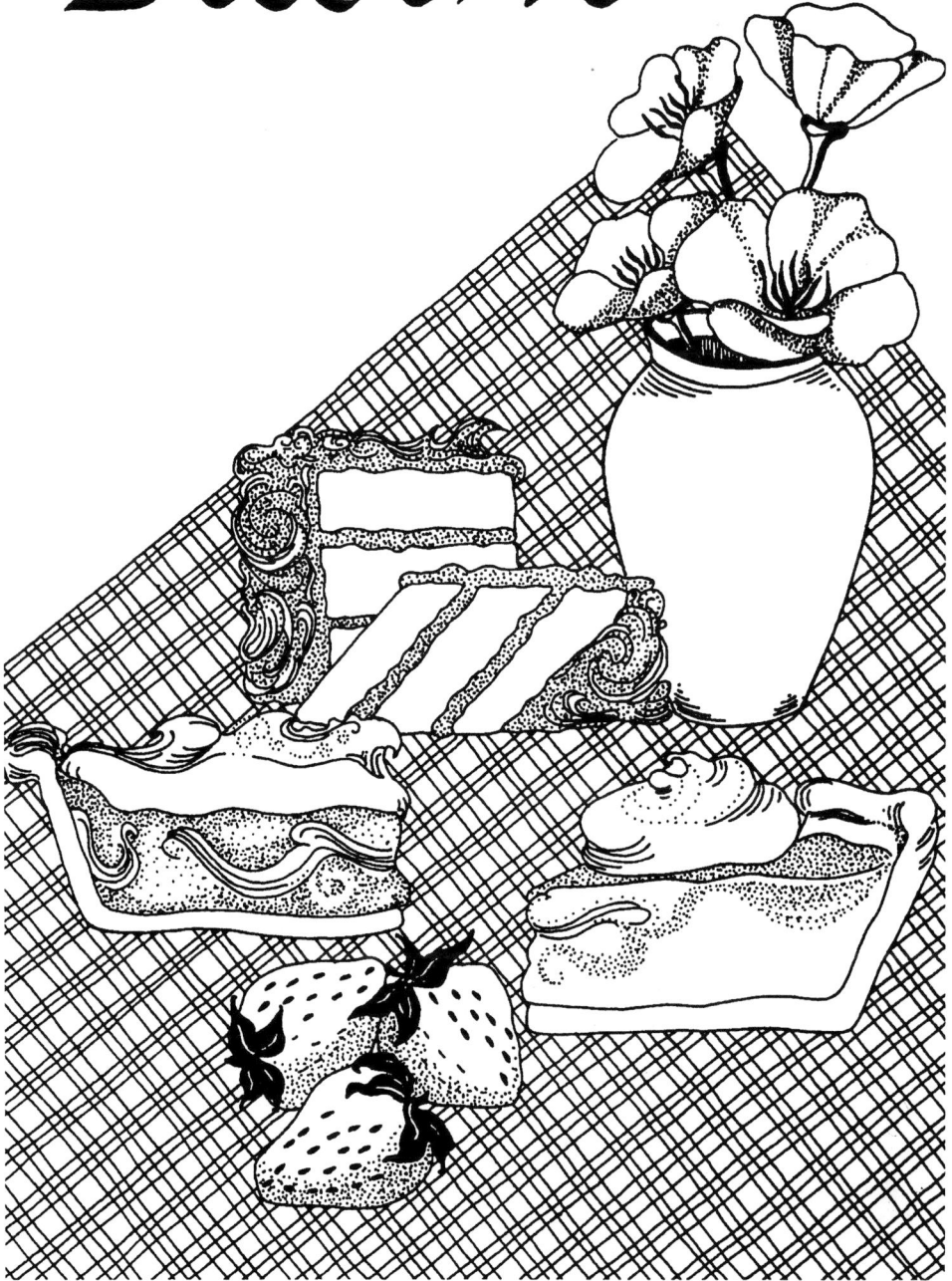

Desserts

Chapter 13

DESSERTS

PUMPKIN PIE*
A Thanksgiving treat

1 1/2 packages Mori Nu Lite® firm tofu
2 cups canned pumpkin
2/3 cup sugar
1 teaspoon vanilla
1 1/2 teaspoons cinnamon
1/4 teaspoon nutmeg
1/4 teaspoon ginger
1 unbaked pastry crust

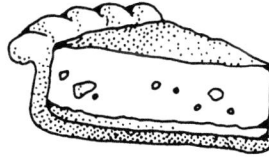

Preheat oven to 350 degrees. Blend tofu in a blender or food processor until smooth. Add remaining ingredients and blend. Pour into a deep pie shell. Bake for 45 minutes.

*See Chapter 14.

SILK PIE
Light and Luscious

1 prebaked pie shell
1/2 cup margarine
1 cup sugar
1 ounce unsweetened non-milk chocolate, melted
1 1/2 tablespoons vanilla
3 eggs or 4 egg whites

Combine all ingredients. Pour into pie shell. Refrigerate for 4 hours or overnight. Top with nondairy whipped cream.

CONNECTICUT TRADITIONAL PUMPKIN PIE
A Yankee Doodle Dandy

1–9 inch unbaked pastry shell
1–16 ounce can pumpkin (2 cups)
1 3/4 cups Farm Fresh Original
1/2 cup sugar
2 eggs
1 teaspoon cinnamon
1/2 teaspoon each ginger, nutmeg, and salt

Preheat oven to 425 degrees. Combine all ingredients except pastry shell. Mix well and pour into pastry shell. Bake 15 minutes. Reduce oven temperature to 350 degrees. Bake 30 to 40 minutes until done. If a knife inserted near the edge comes out clean, it is done. Cool and garnish.

BOSTON CREAM PIE
The Pilgrims missed this one!

Preheat oven to 350 degrees F. Grease or spray 2 round 9-inch cake pans.

1 Betty Crocker® Pound Cake Mix (pareve), prepared according to directions.

To make filling: Use 1-3 ounces *not-instant* vanilla pudding using 2 cups of Farm Rich Non-dairy Creamer (1 part Farm Rich to 1 part water). Cook using directions on package.

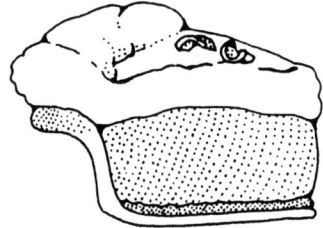

Icing:
1 tablespoon margarine
2 ounces semisweet chocolate-no lactose
1/2 cup powered sugar
2 to 3 tablespoons Farm Rich as prepared above.

Place one cake layer on a plate and spread with pudding. Place a second layer on top. Frost top with icing. Refrigerate until serving time.

SWEET POTATO PIE*
A Southern Delight

1 graham cracker crust (ready-made can be used)
12 ounces firm silken tofu
1-2 tablespoons orange juice
1/4 cup canola oil
1 cup cooked or canned mashed sweet potatoes
1/2 teaspoon cinnamon

Combine all ingredients and pour into graham cracker crust. Bake at 350 degrees for 30-35 minutes.

*See Chapter 14.

LUDLOW GOLDEN SPONGE LOAF
Springy

4 eggs or one container of 4 egg whites substitute.
   Read label on carton–some use dairy products to process.
1 cup sugar
2 tablespoons vegetable oil
2 teaspoons vanilla
2 teaspoons grated orange rind
1 teaspoon baking powder
1/8 teaspoon salt
1 1/2 cups flour

Preheat oven to 350 degrees. Grease or spray 1 loaf pan (8 1/2 x 4 1/2 x 2 1/2). Beat eggs. add sugar, oil, vanilla, and rind. Add salt, baking powder, and flour. Bake 20-24 minutes until golden (hence the name). Drizzle with a nondairy chocolate sauce, or top with strawberries and nondairy whipped topping.

ULTRA LIGHT SOUFFLÉ-LIKE CHOCOLATE CAKE
A Summer's Delight

2 egg whites (or egg whit substitute, 1/2 cup)
1 cup sugar
1/2 cup Hershey's® cocoa powder
2 tablespoons flour
3 tablespoons vegetable oil (not olive oil)
1/4 tsp vanilla
4 fresh egg whites

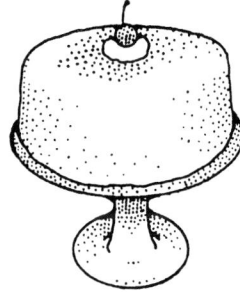

Beat all ingredients together. Beat 4 fresh egg whites until stiff, thoroughly fold into the chocolate mixture. Pour into a lightly greased springform pan with a removable bottom. Bake at 350 degrees for 25 minutes. This cake will puff up and then fall when removed from the pan. That's OK. When cool, sprinkle with confectioner's sugar.

STARS AND STRIPES FOREVER
A "Major" Cake

1 Betty Crocker Pound Cake Mix (pareve)
12 x 8 inch baking dish
1 cup blueberries
3 cups sliced strawberries, halved
1 tub (12oz) nondairy whipped topping

Bake cake mix according to directions. Cool. Line bottom of baking dish with slices of cake. Spread the nondairy topping evenly over the cake. Design a flag by using the 1 cup blueberries "stars" in the upper left corner of the cake. Use the halved strawberries (rounded sides up) to create the "stripes" effect. Refrigerate at least 1-2 hours. Serves 10-12.

MANCHESTER CHOCOLATE DREAM CAKE
A Hint of Orange

2 cups flour
1/2 cup sugar
1/2 cup cocoa
1 1/2 teaspoons baking powder
1/8 teaspoons salt (optional)
1 teaspoon baking soda
2 large eggs
3/4 cup vegetable oil (not olive)
1/2 cup orange juice
1/2 cup cold water
2 teaspoons vanilla

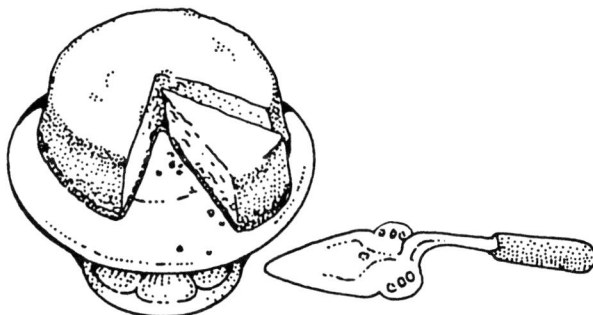

Preheat oven to 350 degrees. Put all dry ingredients into a mixing bowl. Add eggs, orange juice, oil, and vanilla. Beat 2 minutes on medium speed, then 5 minutes on high. Grease or spray a 13 x 9 baking pan. Bake 26-28 minutes. Cool 10 minutes before removing. Frost with a nondairy frosting or whipped topping.

NONDAIRY CHOCOLATE CAKE
Truly scrumptious

2 cups flour
1/2 cup white sugar
1/2 cup Hershey's cocoa
1 1/2 teaspoon baking powder
1/8 teaspoon salt
1 teaspoon baking soda
2 large eggs
3/4 cup vegetable oil (not olive oil)
1/2 cup orange juice
1/2 cup cold water
2 teaspoons vanilla

Preheat oven to 350 degrees. Put dry ingredients in large mixer bowl. Add eggs, juice, and vanilla. Beat 2 minutes on medium speed and 5 minutes on high speed. Lightly grease a 13 x 9 inch metal pan. Bake 26 to 28 minutes. Cool and serve, or freeze for later.

MONDEL BRÜD OR BISCOTTI
In German or Italian, it's delicious

1/4 pound margarine
1 cup sugar
2 eggs
2 cups flour
1 teaspoon baking powder
1 teaspoon vanilla
3/4 cup chopped nuts (your choice–almonds for biscotti)
1/4 cup chocolate bits (optional–make sure no lactose)

Cream margarine and sugar. Add eggs. Add flour, baking powder, nuts, vanilla, and optional chocolate bits. With slightly wet hands, divide batter and form into 4 bars. Place on a greased or sprayed cookie sheet and bake at 350 degrees for 20-25 minutes until golden brown. Cool 10 minutes and remove. When completely cold, cut into slices

*For a mocha taste, add 2 tablespoons instant coffee to batter.

A WINNING DESSERT REDONE
Very Airy

1/4 cup Farm Fresh Original
6 ounces white chocolate chips
1 egg (room temperature)
1 tablespoon instant coffee dissolved in
  2 tablespoons hot water
1/2 teaspoon cinnamon
1 teaspoon vanilla
1/2 cup nondairy whipped topping

Scald Farm Fresh Original. In a blender, place chips, egg, dissolved coffee, cinnamon, and vanilla. While blender is running, add scalded "cream" through the open top of the lid. Remove when blended. Put in a bowl and refrigerate for one-half hour. Fold in whipped topping. Spoon into 6 serving glasses.

BLUEBERRY BREAD PUDDING
Hustle down to the berry patch

2 cups Farm Rich Light or 1 part Farm Rich
   and 3 parts water
1 cup Egg Beaters® egg product
2/3 cup sugar
1 teaspoon vanilla
1/4 teaspoon ground cinnamon
8 slices white bread, cubed (4 cups)
1 cup fresh or frozen blueberries

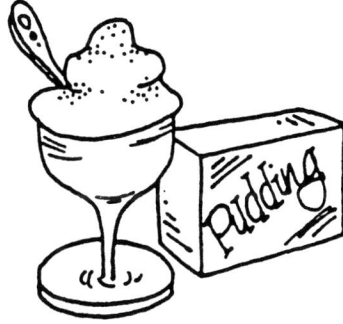

In a large bowl, blend together Farm Rich, Egg Beaters, sugar, vanilla, and cinnamon. Set aside. Place bread cubes in lightly greased or sprayed 8 x 8 x 2 inch baking dish. Sprinkle with blueberries. Pour egg mixture evenly over bread mixture. Set dish in a pan filled with 1 inch depth of hot water. Bake at 350 degrees for 1 hour or until set.

Hint: Try this with raspberries (red or black)

GRAPE-NUTS® PUDDING
Old-Fashioned Favorite

1/2 cup Grape-Nuts cereal
2 cups enriched rice milk or
*1 cup each, Fresh Farm Original and water
2 eggs beaten
1/2 cup sugar
1/2 teaspoon vanilla
dash of nutmeg or cinnamon

Warm rice milk or combination of Farm Fresh Original and water. Pour over Grape-Nuts. Let stand 15 minutes. Add eggs, sugar, and vanilla. Mix well and pour into a greased 9 x 9 x 2 inch baking pan. Sprinkle with nutmeg or cinnamon on top. Place pan in a larger pan with 1 inch of hot water in bottom. Bake 350 degrees for one hour, or until knife inserted in middle comes out clean.

*1 cup Farm Rich® to a cup water.

CHOCOLATE BREAD PUDDING
A nondairy redux. Thanks to The Hartford Courant!

2 ounces baking chocolate
2 cups Farm Rich Skim Nondairy Creamer
1/2 teaspoon salt
1/2 cup brown sugar
nondairy whipped topping (not lite)
1 1/2 teaspoons vanilla
6 slices, dry bread cut into 1/2 inch cubes
handful of walnut pieces
2 eggs

Heat chocolate and Farm Rich in double broiler until chocolate is melted. Add salt. Combine brown sugar and eggs and beat lightly. Add chocolate mixture gradually, stirring vigorously. Stir in vanilla. Combine bread and chocolate mixture. Stir in walnuts if desired. Let mixture stand 10 to 15 minutes. Stir and turn into a greased 1 1/2 quart casserole. Place in a pan of of water and bake 30 minutes at 350 degrees. Cool and garnish with whipped nondairy topping.

RICE PUDDING
A Creamy Touch

1/2 cup uncooked white rice (not instant)
1 quart vanilla enriched Rice Dream milk
1/2 cup sugar
1 teaspoon vanilla
1/8 teaspoon salt
1/2 teaspoon cinnamon

Preheat oven to 325 degrees. Combine rice milk, rice, sugar, vanilla, and salt. Pour into a greased 1 1/2 quart casserole dish. Cover and bake for 2 hours until rice is soft. Remove cover and bake a few minutes longer. Sprinkle with cinnamon and serve.

RASPBERRY TRIFLE
Almost British

1 package Betty Crocker golden pound cake mix
1 package (4-serving size) vanilla pudding
  (not instant)
1 cup orange juice
1/2 cup raspberry preserves
2 cups nondairy whipped cream (or see page 77)
1/4 cup slivered almonds

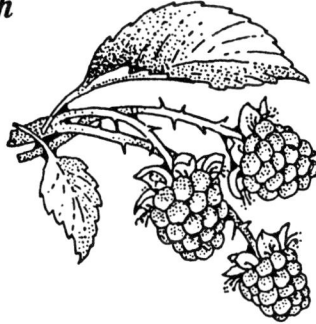

Heat oven to 325 degrees. Grease or spray 2 loaf pans, 8 1/2 x 4 1/2 x 2 1/2. Bake and cool. Freeze 1 loaf for another use, another time.

Prepare pudding using enriched rice milk or lactose reduced milk. Cut remaining loaf into 1-inch cubes. Place half the pieces into a see-through glass bowl. Sprinkle with the orange juice. Spoon half of the preserves over the pieces. Spread with 1 cup of pudding. Repeat for second layer.

Cover and refrigerate for at least 4 hours. To serve, spread with nondairy whipped cream. Sprinkle with almonds and garnish with raspberries.

FRUITY PUDDIN'
Fast and Simple

1–30 ounce can of fruit cocktail
1 egg beaten
1 teaspoon vanilla
1 cup flour
3/4 sugar
1 teaspoon baking soda
1/2 teaspoon salt (optional)
1/2 cup brown sugar
1/2 cup nuts

Combine fruit cocktail and syrup, egg and vanilla. Combine rest of the ingredients and add fruit cocktail mixture. Pour into 9 x 12 greased or sprayed baking pan. Sprinkle with brown sugar and nuts. Bake at 350 degrees for 45 minutes. Top with nondairy whipped cream.

WHIPPED TOPPING*
Made "From Scratch"

10 1/2 ounces firm silken tofu
2-4 tablespoons powdered sugar or to taste
1/4 teaspoons vanilla
1/8 teaspoons salt
soy milk as needed or nondairy milk

Combine all ingredients in blender. Blend until smooth. Add soy milk a little at a time. Place in a covered container and refrigerate until well chilled. Makes 1 3/4 cups.

*See Chapter 14.

PIZZA FOR DESSERT?
Let the kids help

1 roll refrigerated cookie dough (no milk solids)
2 cups thawed Cool Whip® Whipped Topping
  (read label-not "lite")
2 cups assorted fruit, cut up (bananas, kiwi,
  strawberries, grape halves, canned or
  fresh peaches, etc.)

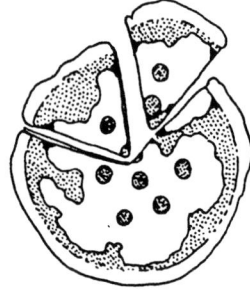

Heat oven to 350 degrees. Press dough into 12-inch pizza pan. Bake 20 minutes until brown. Cool in pan. Carefully lift out of pan. Place cookie crust on serving plate. Spread whipped topping on cookie crust. Garnish withe the cut-up fruit. To serve, cut in wedges like a pizza. Mangia!

APRICOT WHIP
Try this one on Guests

1 1/2 cups dried apricots
1/2 cup sugar
1 cup Cool Whip nondairy topping (not "lite")

Bring apricots to a boil and simmer 20 minutes. Cool. Place apricots and sugar in blender and blend for 20 seconds. Fold in Cool Whip. Spoon into sherbet glasses.

NONDAIRY ICE CREAM
Can you believe it?

3 egg whites
1/2 cup sugar
8 ounces nondairy whipped topping–check label
  (not "lite")
3 egg yolks
1 teaspoon vanilla
2 tablespoons flavorings of your choice: almond,
  rum, chocolate peppermint extract, or berries

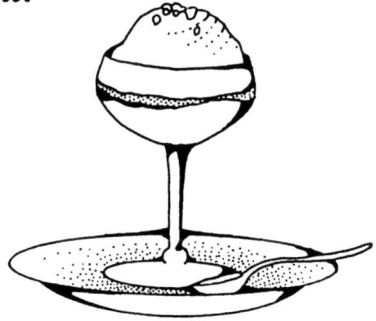

Separate eggs. Whip egg whites with 1/4 cup sugar until lemon colored. Blend the yolks and vanilla into the whipped topping. Fold the egg white mixture (meringue) into this mixture. Add flavorings or fruit. Freeze until firm.

COCOA FREEZE
Summer Kid's Play

1 cup Farm Rich nondairy creamer
1/2 cup Cool Whip nondairy topping
1 tablespoon cocoa powder

Mix ingredients together in a blender, or beat vigorously with a wire whip. Pout into a bowl and freeze overnight. Spoon into dishes and top with nondairy topping.

CHOCOLATE MOUSSE*
Tofu is the secret

1/2 cup enriched vanilla Rice Dream nondairy beverage
1 tablespoon orange juice concentrate
1 1/4 cups Baker's® chocolate chips
1 teaspoon vanilla extract
1/4 teaspoon almond extract
1–10.5 ounce package firm silken tofu.

Warm Rice Dream and orange juice concentrate in a heavy sauce pan. Bring to a simmer and stir in chocolate chips. Remove from heat and stir until the chips are melted and mixture is smooth. Put extracts and tofu in a blender and blend until well-mixed. Chill at least 2 hours. Serve with nondairy whipped topping if desired.

*See Chapter 14.

SORBET

The original Turkish word "sharab" was used to describe a soft, sweet drink. It was replaced by "sorbet" and "sherbet." Another word in English that is derived from the original word is "syrup."

For lactose intolerant sweet lovers, remember that sorbet is made from fruit and ices and contains no dairy products. However, sherbet is made with milk.

VERY BERRY SORBET
Tropical Delight

1 pound any kind of berries
1 cup sugar
1-2 cups water, depending on how juicy berries are
3 tablespoons fruit flavored liqueur (optional)
1 lemon (juice only)
1 orange (juice only)

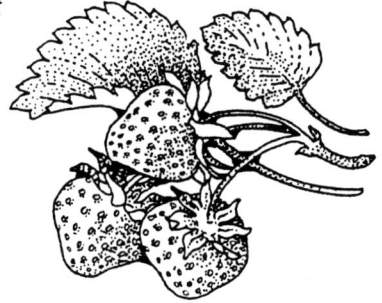

Simmer the water and sugar in pan for five minutes. Cool and then add lemon and orange juice (approximately 1 tablespoon each). Puree berries in a blender and then gradually add the sugar and water syrup. If you use liqueur, add it last. Put mixture into a covered plastic bowl and place in the freezer. Stir after 2 or 3 hours and return to freezer. Stir every half hour until texture is smooth like sherbet. Spoon into serving glasses. Serves 6 to 8.

CRANBERRY SORBET
"A Pilgram's Gift"

1–32 ounce bottle cranberry juice cocktail
2 cups fresh cranberries
1 1/4 cups sugar
2 tablespoons lemon juice

Boil cranberries and cranberry juice uncovered for 5 minutes until the skins on the cranberries pop. Press mixture through a sieve or ricer. Discard skins. Stir in sugar and lemon juice. Pour into a 2-quart baking dish. Freeze 6 hours until firm. Stir every hour. Scoop into a serving dish.

TEN MINUTE PEACH SORBET*
The secret is in the can.

1–16 ounce can sliced or halved peaches in
  heavy syrup

Freeze unopened can of fruit until frozen
solid, at least 18 hours. Submerge
unopened can in hot water 1 to 2 minutes.
Open can and pour syrup into food
processor bowl. Remove other end of can
and turn fruit onto a cutting surface. Cut
into 1 inch slices, then into chunks and
add to processor bowl, pulsating, on and
off, until smooth. Serve immediately or
spoon into a bowl, cover and freeze until
ready to serve–up to 8 hours. Makes 1
1/2 cups of sorbet.

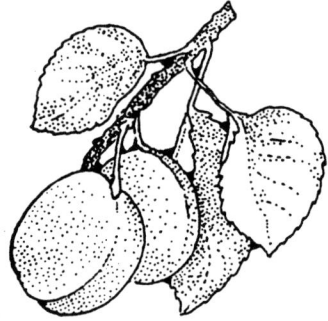

If you care to use a liqueur, add 2 tablespoons during the processing.

Try this with other canned fruits using lemon juice as a flavor
enhancer.

Note: Using a blender makes the recipe too icy. The can may bulge
slightly during freezing, but that's OK.

*Thanks to Melanie Barnard for this creation.

CANTALOUPE ICE
REFRESHING

3 cups pureed cantaloupe (1 large ripe melon)
2 tablespoons lemon or lime juice
1 cup dry white wine or 1 cup white grape juice
2/3 cup sugar
1 cup water

Boil together sugar and water in a saucepan until the sugar is dissolved. Set aside to cool. Mix the puree with the sugar syrup, lemon juice, and wine or grape juice and pour through a wire sieve into a bowl. Freeze for several hours, stirring occasionally to mix frozen crystals. Just before serving, fluff with a fork and spoon into wine glasses or sherbet cups. Serves 6.

CAPPUCCINO MIX*
A Continental treat

1 cup nondairy coffee creamer
1 cup nondairy chocolate drink mix (Nestles Quik®)
2/3 cup coffee crystals
1/2 cup sugar
1/2 teaspoon ground cinnamon

Store in an air tight container. To prepare one serving, add 1 1/2 - 2 tablespoons of mix to 6 ounces of hot water. This recipe makes 3 cups of dry mix.

*Courtesy of *The Hartford Courant.*

CREAMY ORANGE JULIUS
A Summer's Delight

1–6 ounce can frozen concentrated orange juice
1 cup 100% Lactaid milk (100% lactose reduced)
　　or Enriched Rice Dream
1 cup water
1 teaspoon vanilla
10 ice cubes
1/4 cup sugar

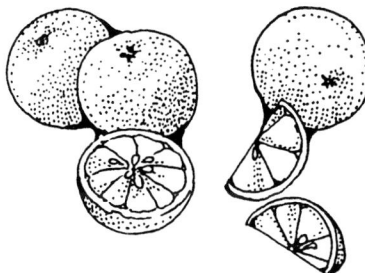

Combine all ingredients in a blender and process 30 seconds or until ice cubes are crushed.

CAROB SHAKE
Super Variation

1 cup Enriched Rice Dream rice milk
2 frozen bananas
2 teaspoons maple syrup
1 tablespoon unsweetened carob powder

Combine all ingredients in a blender and blend until smooth.

AMBROSIA SHAKE
Fit for the Gods!

2 ripe bananas
2-3 tablespoons orange juice
2 tablespoons sugar
1/4 teaspoon almond or vanilla extract
1 cup soy milk, or enriched rice milk, or Lactaid 100% lactose reduced milk

Combine all ingredients in a blender and blend for 20 seconds.

MOUSSE AU CHOCOLATE
Rich and Delicious

2 eggs
1 tablespoon sugar
1 tablespoon instant coffee or coffee liqueur
6 ounces semi-sweet, lactose-free chocolate chips (do not melt)
3/4 cup hot, but not boiling, Farm Rich fat-free nondairy creamer

Mix all ingredients together in the blender for 20-40 seconds at high speed. Chill thoroughly. This recipe serves 4 in dessert dishes, or you can use the mousse as a filling for cakes or pies.

RICE DREAM SMOOTHIE
Georgia Special

1/2 ripe banana peeled, frozen and cut into chunks
1 cup chocolate flavored Rice Dream
1/2 teaspoon vanilla
1 tablespoon smooth peanut butter

Blend together until smooth and frothy.

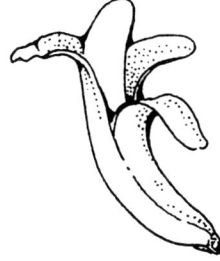

HOT CHOCOLATE
Try this "Apres Ski"

1 1/2 ounces unsweetened chocolate
2 cups hot enriched rice milk
1/4 cup sugar
dash salt

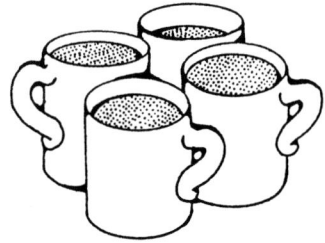

Chop chocolate in blender container for 9 seconds. Add sugar and milk and dash of salt. Cover and turn motor on low for 5 seconds, then on high for 15 seconds. Pour into cups.

MICROWAVE PEANUT BRITTLE
Land's End Easy and Best Candy by Joan C.

1 cup dry roasted-peanuts–not salted
1/2 cup corn syrup
1/8 teaspoon salt
1 cup sugar
1 teaspoon margarine
1 teaspoon vanilla
1 teaspoon baking soda

Stir corn syrup, salt, peanuts, and sugar together in a 1 1/2 quart bowl. Microwave on high for 4 minutes. Stir. Microwave another 3 minutes on high. Add margarine and vanilla. Microwave on high for 1-2 minutes or until caramel colored. Add baking soda and pour onto a greased cookie sheet. Cool well. Break apart and store in an air-tight container.

QUINCY, MASSACHUSETTS ALMOND BUTTERCRUNCH
*A Holiday Favorite**

2 sticks margarine
3/4 cup sugar
unsalted saltines
1–12 ounce bag chocolate chips (nondairy)
sliced almonds

In a saucepan, bring the margarine and sugar to a boil. Line a cookie sheet (with sides) or 2, 11 x 14 inch baking pans with heavy duty aluminum foil and grease the foil with margarine. Line the foil with a single layer of saltines. Pour the margarine and sugar mixture over the crackers and spread evenly. Place in a 400 degree oven for 5 minutes. Remove and sprinkle with the chocolate chips. Return pan to oven for 1 minute to melt. Spread chocolate evenly and top with sliced almonds. Refrigerate to harden. Break or cut into pieces.

*During the Passover holiday season, substitute sheets of Matzos (not egg type) for the saltines.

Chapter 14

NOW, A WORD ABOUT TOFU

Tofu or soybean curd is a valuable, complete protein product of delicate cheese-like consistency that is processed from hot soy milk. Tofu is a totally lactose-free product that can be used to create wonderful recipes or adapted for use as an alternative to dairy products.

Although tofu has a bland, slightly sweet flavor, it easily absorbs the flavors of the other ingredients and seasoning in recipes. It is a staple of Asian cuisines such as Chinese, Vietnamese, Indonesian, and Thai. Vegetarians have known for many years the benefits of cooking with tofu.

Tofu packed in water will last about two weeks unopened, in the refrigerator. However, once open, continue to store any left over tofu in water, but rinse the tofu and replace with fresh water every other day. Soft tofu is best for salad dressings, dips, puddings, or any food with a soft texture. Firm tofu has a chewier texture and can be used in stir-fry and stews. Try experimenting with tofu—you will probably be pleased to find out more of what you can do with it and how to take the mystery out of this remarkable food.

Chapter 15

CONVERSION CHART

Farm Rich/Coffee Rich Nondairy Creamer Conversion Chart

	Farm Rich	*Farm Rich Light*
heavy cream or half & half	equal amounts	does not apply
whole milk	1 part Farm Rich 1 part water	equal amount
skim milk	1 part Farm Rich 3 parts water	1 part Farm Rich Light & 1 part water

Farm Rich/Coffee Rich®, Nondairy Creamers are interchangeable in their uses in recipe preparation. These products contain no lactose and can be used as a substitute for dairy milk or cream. They are kosher and pareve.

There are other brands of nondairy creamers that can be used. Read ingredients carefully.

BIBLIOGRAPHY

Goodman, R.M. *Genetic Disorders Among Jewish People.* Johns Hopkins University Press, Baltimore and London, 1979.

Diamond, Harvey & Marilyn Diamond. *Fit for Life, Living Healthy.* Warner Books Inc., New York.

Rosenfeld, I., *Doctor, What Should I Eat?* Random House, New York.

INDEX

101

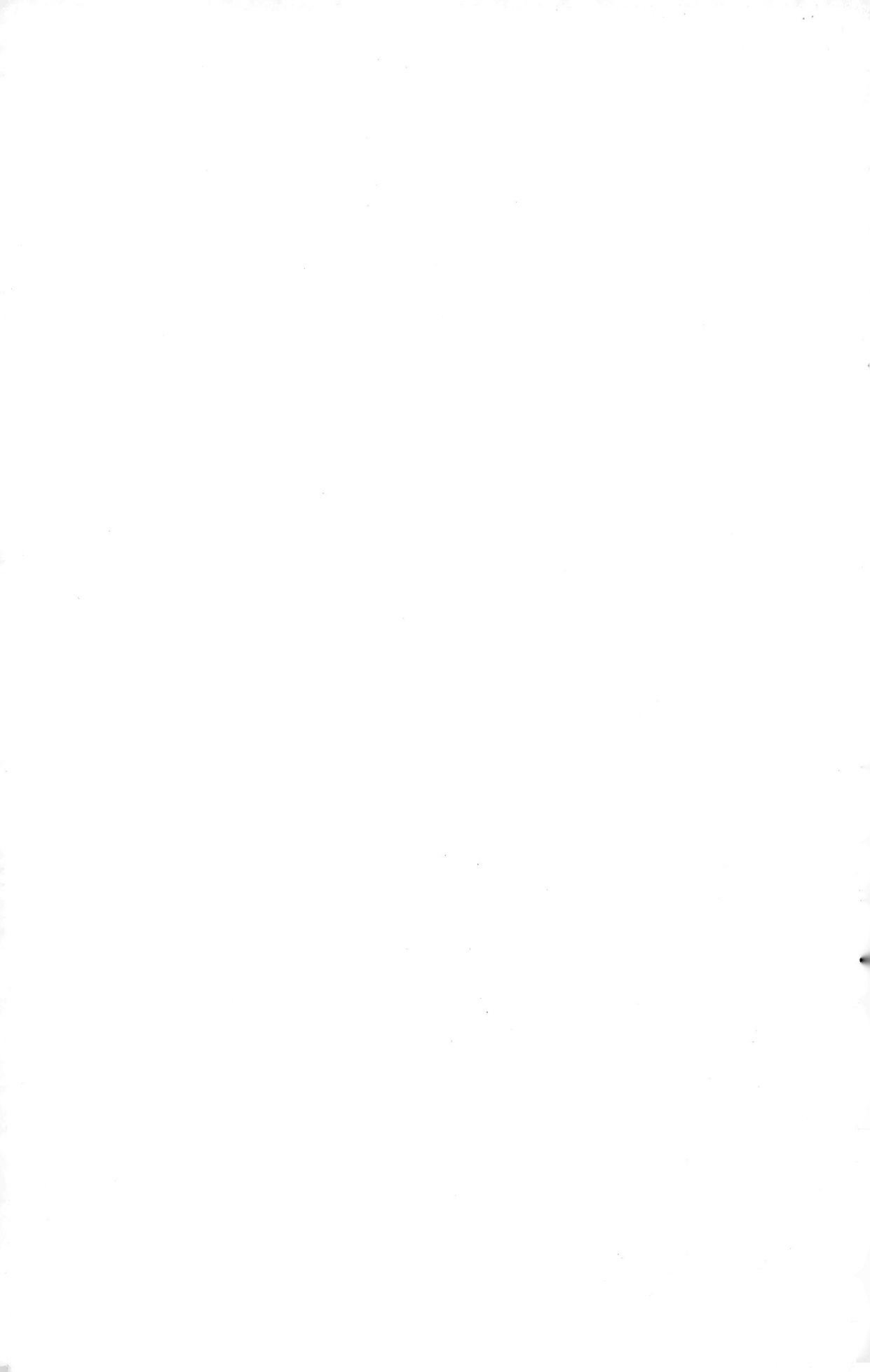